Understanding Schizophrenia

Causes, cures, and how to live with schizophrenia

Table of Contents

Introduction iv

Chapter 1 – Introduction to Schizophrenia 1

Chapter 2 – The Onset of Schizophrenia 4

Chapter 3 – Schizophrenia: Signs and Symptoms 7

Chapter 4 – Causes and Specific Symptoms Based on the Different Types of Schizophrenia 11

Chapter 5 – Living with Schizophrenia 15

Chapter 6 – Coping with Schizophrenia: Family and Sufferer 18

Conclusion 21

Introduction

I want to thank you and congratulate you for downloading the book, *"Understanding Schizophrenia"*.

This book contains helpful information on what causes schizophrenia and how this condition works.

There are several types of schizophrenia, each of which is explained in depth in the following chapters.

You will soon learn exactly what it means to be a schizophrenic, and will discover many myths about schizophrenia that are simply untrue.

While there is no definitive cure for schizophrenia as yet, there are several treatment options available. With the right treatment and support, a schizophrenic will have the best chance of leading a normal and positive life.

Further in this book, you will learn how schizophrenia can be treated, and the role that families and friends can play in the treatment process.

The aim of this book is to explain to you techniques and tips for fighting against schizophrenia, and to help you better understand the condition.

Thanks again for downloading this book, I hope you enjoy it!

Chapter 1 – Introduction to Schizophrenia

Schizophrenia is a serious mental illness that affects over two million Americans. While there are a lot of misconceptions about this very challenging and serious medical condition, it can be treated. However, if the condition is left untreated, it can create a major impact on the lives of the people suffering the disease and their families.

What is Schizophrenia?

Schizophrenia is a mental illness characterized by psychosis. It's a mysterious brain disorder that creates a different perception of reality. It distorts the way one thinks, expresses emotions, acts, and relates towards other people. This is considered to be the most debilitating of all of the recognized mental illnesses. It creates problems in a person's relationships at home, at work, at school, and in society in general. Luckily, this life-long illness can be treated and controlled.

People who are diagnosed with schizophrenia often see and hear things that do not really exist. They are often seen speaking in confusing ways. Most of the time they feel paranoia that there are people who are trying to harm them, or they have a feeling of being watched at all times.

Debunking the Myths

There are many myths that go around about schizophrenia. Below are some of the common ones, along with the explanations of what being schizophrenic really means.

Myth #1: Patients with schizophrenia have multiple personalities (split personality disorder).

Fact #1: Multiple personality disorder is a different illness all-together. It is less common compared to schizophrenia. Schizophrenics do not have multiple personalities, but rather they see a different reality.

Myth #2: Only a few people can get schizophrenia.

Fact #2: This illness is not rare; in fact, doctors say that 1 in 1000 people are likely to develop schizophrenia.

Myth #3: Schizophrenics are dangerous people.

Fact #3: Patients may be characterized as delusional, and may experience hallucinations, but they are not as dangerous as what others perceive them to be. Although there are some patients who may exhibit violent behavior, they are more dangerous to themselves than to others.

Myth #4: There is no hope for people suffering from schizophrenia.

Fact #4: Schizophrenia can be treated. However, the treatment takes time. With proper diagnosis and treatment, the patient can live a normal life.

Myth #5: Schizophrenics are not capable of making decisions on their own and they need their family to decide things for them.

Fact #5: When a person is diagnosed with schizophrenia, it doesn't mean that the patient will be dependent on their family for everything. What most people don't realize is that patients diagnosed with schizophrenia can handle their own affairs with very little or no help at all. There can be cases, however, where patients experience symptoms that hinder them from making decisions. In these instances they may need someone to step in to help for a short time.

Chapter 2 – The Onset of Schizophrenia

When you have schizophrenia, your ability to think clearly, make decisions, and manage your emotions is significantly impaired. Most of those who have schizophrenia suffer from delusions and hallucinations. The disease has been linked to changes in the brain's chemistry and structure. This is a very complex mental health condition that affects people in a variety of different ways.

The onset of the disease in most patients is gradual and occurs mostly in early adulthood, usually in the early 20's. Most of the time, a patient's family and friends fail to recognize the early symptoms that can manifest before the primary symptoms occur.

During the initial stages of schizophrenia, a person may not have set goals in life. They often become unmotivated and tend to withdraw socially, to the point of becoming eccentric and reclusive, even from family and friends. They begin to exhibit a feeling of indifference to life. However, in some patients, the illness appears without warning. Its severity varies from one patient to another.

These are the most common signs that can be manifested at the onset of schizophrenia:

- Social withdrawal
- Paranoia
- Increase unfounded suspiciousness
- Hostility, especially towards criticism

- Deterioration of personal hygiene
- Inability to express emotions
- Depression
- Expressionless gaze
- Uttering irrational statements
- Oversleeping or insomnia
- Deterioration of personal hygiene
- Odd or bizarre beliefs
- Lack of motivation
- Reliance on drugs and/or alcohol

Doctors say that these signs can indicate a lot of other possible medical problems, but can potentially indicate schizophrenia. This is often true for people who experience continuous deterioration in their behaviors and actions.

Subtypes of Schizophrenia

Schizophrenia is actually a term that refers to a complex group of mental illnesses. However, most of its subtypes show similar signs and symptoms.

Here are the different types of schizophrenia in relation to the symptoms:

- **Paranoid schizophrenia**

Those who have paranoid schizophrenia are mostly preoccupied with false beliefs or delusions that they are punished or persecuted by other people.

- **Disorganized schizophrenia**

With disorganized schizophrenia, patients are confused. They often exhibit jumbled speech and become extremely incoherent. They have the tendency to become emotionally flat. They find it hard to show emotions, and sometimes become inappropriate in their actions and behaviors, to the point of being childlike. Their disorganized behavior often causes disruption to their everyday activities.

- **Catatonic schizophrenia**

People with catatonic schizophrenia have more obvious physical symptoms of the illness.

- **Undifferentiated schizophrenia**

This refers to the type of schizophrenia that has symptoms that do not clearly point to the condition.

- **Residual schizophrenia**

The severity of the symptoms in residual schizophrenia is markedly decreased. The delusions and hallucinations are still observed but they are less manifested. There will be an evidence of disturbing behaviors which might include blank looks, lack of interest in the people around them, monotone speech, and expressionless faces.

In the next chapter, you will learn more about the signs, symptoms, and causes of the disease.

Chapter 3 – Schizophrenia: Signs and Symptoms

People with schizophrenia may show several symptoms that involve extreme changes in their behaviors and their personality in general. During the early stages of the illness, the symptoms often appear suddenly.

The most common causes of the illness can be divided into three categories, namely, positive, negative, and disorganized symptoms.

The Positive Symptoms

Positive here doesn't mean they are "good" symptoms, it simply means that these symptoms are not seen in people that do not have the illness. They are also often called psychotic symptoms:

- *Delusions*
  Delusions are strange or false beliefs of events and situations. These beliefs are not based on reality. For instance, the patient may have been roused from sleep because of the noise made by neighbors, and they immediately jump to the conclusion that this was a deliberate attempt to disturb them in their sleep. They often have the belief that the people who make suspicious looks toward them are plotting something bad against them.

  People who exhibit delusionary symptoms tend to personalize everything that happens around them. They also don't back down with their false beliefs, even when presented with factual evidence or information disproving their belief.

Lots of the time, before being diagnosed, families and friends will simply think that the patient is just stubborn or stupid. Patients' delusions can become irritating to the people hearing them, especially if they hear them often.

Delusions occur in over 90% of patients with schizophrenia. These delusions often involve illogical ideas. Doctors identified the following common delusions:

- **Delusions of persecution** – These involve the belief of schizophrenics that other people are out to "get them". These patients often have bizarre plots that they have concocted.

- **Delusions of reference** – Patients with schizophrenia often believe that they are incarnates, or they are actually famous people or important figures in the history of mankind, like Christopher Columbus or even Jesus. Sometimes they believe that they have superhero powers.

- **Delusions of control** – Those who have delusions of control often believe that there is an outside force, like an alien, that controls their actions and thoughts. They usually believe that their own thoughts are being sent to other people.

- *Hallucinations*
Hallucinations are characterized by false perceptions that often affect a patient's senses. People exhibiting

hallucinations often see, hear, taste, smell, and touch something that is not really there. These people often insist that they keep hearing voices in their heads, but not a single person around them can hear these voices.

Some patients experience more obvious symptoms. Most of the time, these voices actually come from their environment. Patients often hear conversations between people and they begin hearing these conversations over and over in their heads.

Still, there are some who believe that these voices in their head are something of supernatural origin. Patients believe that these voices are real and not just their wild imagination working.

- *Catatonia*
  Catatonia is characterized when a person becomes fixated in a single posture or position for a very long period of time.

Negative Schizophrenic Symptoms

The negative symptoms refer to the nonexistence of the usual behaviors found in healthy individuals. These include the following:

- ***Absence of emotional expression*** – A normal person will usually react to things and the people around them. A person with schizophrenia usually exhibits an inexpressive or blank face, avoids eye contact, and talks in a flat voice.

- ***Lack of enthusiasm*** – The schizophrenic patient has lackluster enthusiasm; they aren't motivated by anything.

- ***Apparent lack of interest in the world around them*** – An individual diagnosed with schizophrenia tends to withdraw from the community. There is usually a total unawareness or lack of interest in the environment and the world they live in.

Disorganized Symptoms and Behaviors

When one has schizophrenia, their goal-directed activity is disrupted, thus hindering their ability to take care of their needs and interact with other people. Disorganized schizophrenic behaviors include:

- Patients are observed to give inappropriate responses
- Marked decline on how they function in their daily activities
- Evident lack of self-control
- Impulsive behaviors
- Tendency to have bizarre behaviors and act without a particular purpose
- There are patients who incessantly write vague words
- Tendency to forget people and things and lose items
- Tendency to repeat actions and gestures, like non-stop walking in circles

In the next chapter, you will learn about the signs and symptoms that can be observed that are specific to different types of schizophrenia.

Chapter 4 – Causes and Specific Symptoms Based on the Different Types of Schizophrenia

Before discussing the symptoms of the illness, it is important that you understand the possible causes of the illness. While doctors have not found its exact cause, studies and tests show that schizophrenia can be the result of the complexity in the interaction between one's genetics and the environment.

Genetics

Schizophrenia has long been linked to one's genetic makeup. Those who have a first degree relative, like a parent or a sibling, who suffers from the illness have a 10% possibility of developing schizophrenia. It has to be noted, however, that the condition is only influenced by the genes one has and not necessarily determined by them. Researches show that while the disease may run in the family, there are about 60% of patients suffering from schizophrenia who do not have other family members afflicted by it. Also, there are individuals considered to be included in the high risk group who do not develop the illness at all.

Environment

Studies show that your genes make you vulnerable to developing schizophrenia, and consequently, your environment exploits that vulnerability that can trigger development of the disease. A common environmental factor is stress. Other environmental factors include:

- Prenatal exposure to infection
- Low oxygen levels at birth
- Exposure to virus at infancy
- Early separation from parents
- Abuse, both physical and sexual, during childhood

Signs and Symptoms

Paranoid Schizophrenia

People with paranoid schizophrenia create stories in their head that they tell consistently over time. The story is often that somebody or a group of people want to inflict harm on them. Their delusions of persecution become more frequent but the story remains the same.

Those patients who have paranoid schizophrenia find it difficult to trust others, even their closest friends and family, thus straining their relationships. However, patients who have developed this subtype of schizophrenia function better in their daily activities compared to those who have a different diagnosis. Their thoughts and actions are more organized and they show better prognosis.

Disorganized Schizophrenia

These people are generally immobile, and mostly unresponsive to the goings around them. They become stiff and extremely unwilling to move. These people are often seen to be assuming bizarre positions and movements. The people around them observe that they have the tendency to repeat words or phrases just spoken by another person. They also have the tendency to become restless and engage in activities that have no specific purpose or specific result, like walking in a straight line going back and forth.

They are likely to become malnourished and often complain of exhaustion. They are also the ones who have the highest risk of inflicting self-injury. They are also likely to suffer from delusions and hallucinations, but their stories are not as consistent as those with paranoid schizophrenia.

Development is gradual. Further manifestations include:

- Communication skills impairment
- Emotional indifference
- Illogical speech
- Peculiar mannerisms
- Inappropriate reactions, like laughing at a funeral

Catatonic Schizophrenia

Individuals with catatonic schizophrenia either show a decrease or an increase in their motor activities.

- **Stuporous state** – Characterized by a reduction in activities. The patient may cease all voluntary speech and movement. They are often resistant to changes in position.

- **Excited state** – Most patients show an episode of extreme excitement. During this episode, they may be heard shouting or talking rapidly. They may also walk non-stop, back and forth. Some even exhibit violent behaviors, making them quite dangerous to themselves and to others.

Patients are more likely to obey commands or mimic what other people say.

Now that you know the symptoms, could you be at risk or do you have a family member or a friend suffering from schizophrenia? Learn more about how to deal and live with schizophrenia in the succeeding chapters.

Chapter 5 – Living with Schizophrenia

When people ignore the symptoms of schizophrenia, or if patients don't get the needed medical attention, the effects of the disorder are adverse not just to the patients, but also to the people around them. The symptoms can result in the following:

- **Strained relationships** – Relationships are bound to suffer due to the disruptions in patients' daily functioning. Their delusions and hallucinations prevent them from acting 'normal' around other people.

- **Disruption in the normal activities** – The disorder deters sufferers from performing their normal everyday functions. Their delusions and hallucinations prevent them from restoring normalcy into their lives.

- **Alcohol and substance abuse** – Many sufferers develop addiction to alcohol and drugs due to the lure of self-medication and/or to relieve symptoms. They are also more likely to become chain smokers.

- **Suicidal tendencies** – They are at high risk of becoming suicidal. Hearing suicidal innuendos from sufferers should not be dismissed, because they can be likely to do as they say during psychotic episodes and in times of depression.

Being aware of the symptoms and the possible effects of schizophrenia, and helping loved ones or getting help for yourself is vital.

Early Diagnosis

The disorder doesn't occur unexpectedly. When a sufferer has schizophrenia, the decline in their normal functioning is gradual. If family members look closely enough, they will be able to detect the early warning signs of the disorder. Early symptoms are common, though not as pronounced as when the disorder is in the more advanced stage. The most important key to detecting the symptoms is the increased awareness of the sudden changes in an individual's behaviors and actions.

Treatment

Schizophrenia is considered to be a life-long condition. There is no cure for the disorder, but it can be managed. The success of treatment depends on the individual's determination and willingness, plus the support and understanding of family and friends.

- *Psychotherapy*

    This is not considered by doctors to be the best treatment for schizophrenia, but it can be used alongside an effective medication regimen. Psychotherapy may include advice, reassurance, and education for proper management of the disorder. Rehabilitation therapy can be helpful to sufferers who are starting to deteriorate in their communication and motor skills.

- ***Medications***

  Schizophrenia, being a complex disorder, is considered to be a mix of thought, mood, and anxiety disorders. Medications include antipsychotic, anti-anxiety, and antidepressant drugs. These drugs downplay the occurrence of hallucinations and delusions. Some medications have side effects, hence many sufferers discontinue taking them regularly.

Chapter 6 – Coping with Schizophrenia: Family and Sufferer

People suffering from schizophrenia have to deal with the stigma of being afflicted with a mental illness. Sufferers often face significant challenges in terms of their relationships with their family and friends. It's important that the family and friends of the sufferer are supporting during the diagnosis and treatment of the condition.

Sufferers need all the support they can get from their family and friends. The situation might be hard to understand, but the last thing that patients with schizophrenia need is to be left to battle this difficult and complex mental disorder alone.

Having a strong support system helps patients to cope with the disorder. One of the most important things to keep in mind is that this disorder is not rare; and as a result, families can get professional support from many different sources.

It pays to be educated. The first step should be to learn about the illness. With a lot of misconceptions about schizophrenia, knowing more about it is very important. It is hard to deal with something that you know very little about. This book is a great place to begin.

Here are some helpful tips for the family and friends of schizophrenics:

- One family member should take the lead for the family, and should be speaking up about the illness.

Patients, when confronted by doctors during assessment and diagnosis, often have trouble opening up about their condition and what they actually feel because most of them are in the denial stage, or they are just simply ignoring the changes that are occurring. If they can communicate their feelings and fears with a family member, this person can pass on the information to the doctors and medical staff.

- Making sure that the patient is complying with the treatment instructions even after being discharged from the hospital is critical. The family should strictly monitor the patient.

- Aside from proper treatment, patients with schizophrenia need emotional support as they continue with their medication regime. Patients have an increased likelihood of falling into depression because of their condition. When they don't get the emotional support they need, they are even more likely to develop depression and anxiety, which can worsen their schizophrenia.

- Family and friends must be well-educated on how to deal with patients when they become delusional and begin to express bizarre beliefs and statements. They should know what to do when patients come up with imaginary situations and events. Some people tend to go along with the delusions, but doctors do not recommend this. Instead, the patient's family should tell the sufferer outright that they do not agree with their assumptions.

    However, care must be undertaken so as not to challenge a schizophrenic's beliefs because for a sufferer, their hallucinations and delusions are their own reality. Arguments will not be helpful. The best thing to do is to divert the sufferer's attention by changing the conversation topic.

- Sufferers need patience and understanding. It will not help them if their own families and friends abandon and disown them. They will struggle to cope with the disorder on their own, and the best support system for patients should come from their loved ones.

- Families should help the sufferer set attainable goals. They need proper encouragement. Families shouldn't make sufferers feel that they are hopeless. By helping them set goals that are simple yet attainable, it helps them get back on track; plus setting something that can be achieved will help unburden them. They can improve their confidence by achieving small goals to start.

- The best way to support your loved ones who have schizophrenia is not to condemn them or make them feel inferior. They are in their lowest point, their confidence levels are down, and they feel hopeless. If you really want to help your loved one to cope with the disorder, you must be there for them.

There may not be a perfect cure for schizophrenia yet, but there are treatments available to make sufferers' lives as normal as possible. With the help of their families and friends, schizophrenics can lead a normal life for a very long time. Hopefully with medical advancements, this condition will eventually be curable, but for now, a good treatment plan is the best option.

Conclusion

Thank you again for downloading this book!

I hope this book was able to help you learn more about schizophrenia.

Whether you personally suffer from schizophrenia, or a family member or friend is afflicted, remember to stay positive and stick to your treatment plan.

Schizophrenia doesn't have to be debilitating. With the right help it can be managed quite effectively.

The next step is to put this information to use, and begin fighting back against schizophrenia.

Finally, if you enjoyed this book, please take the time to share your thoughts and post a review on Amazon. It'd be greatly appreciated!

Thank you and good luck!

www.ingramcontent.com/pod-product-compliance
Lightning Source LLC
LaVergne TN
LVHW021750060526
838200LV00052B/3573